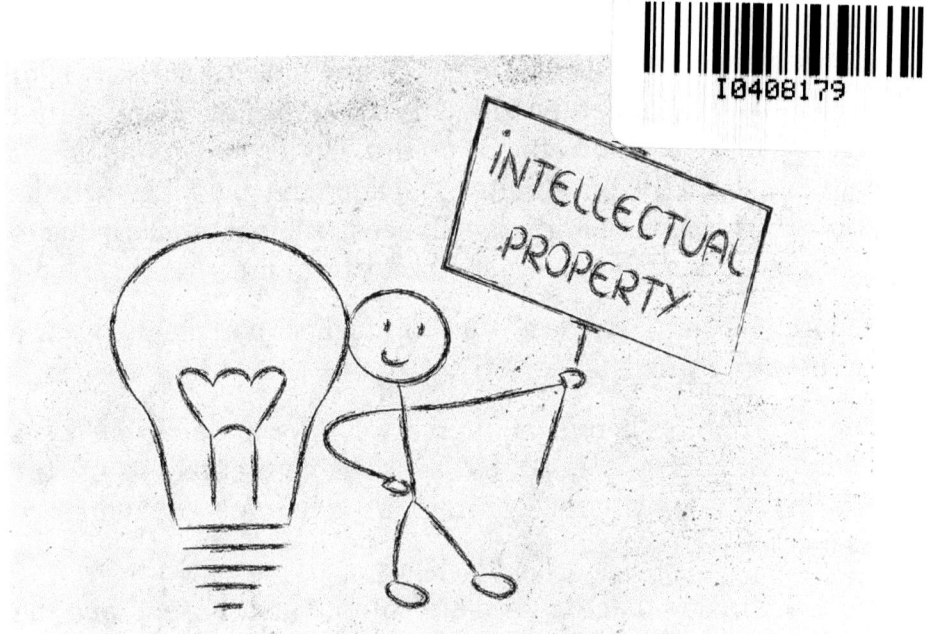

This document is geared toward providing exact and reliable information in regard to the topic and issue covered. The publication is sold with the idea that the publisher is not required to render accounting, officially permitted, or otherwise, qualified services. If advice is necessary, legal or professional, a practiced individual in the profession should be ordered.

- From a Declaration of Principles which was accepted and approved equally by a Committee of the American Bar Association and a Committee of Publishers and Associations.

The information provided herein is stated to be truthful and consistent, in that any liability, in terms of inattention or

Table of Contents

Prevalence of the diet, its decline, and re-emergence

Although the ketogenic diet was discovered in the 1920's for the treatment of pediatric epilepsy, its use in the treatment of this and other debilitating diseases such as convulsive seizures suffered a setback when effective medicines came into the limelight a decade later. These anti-convulsion medicines proved to be easier to implement since the ketogenic diet was difficult to acquire while the world was at war. However, in the mid-1990s, an American movie producer called Jim Abrahams reintroduced it as an effective alternative after it assisted his son recover from serious epilepsy. However, the diet still comes under immense criticism based on its adverse side effects that range from constipation to kidney stones in serious cases. While some dieticians have modified it into the Adkin's diet to reduce these problems, the diet remains highly effective against stubborn cases of epilepsy especially among younger patients.

What is the ketogenic diet?

The ketogenic diet is an isocaloric diet rich in fat and very low in carbohydrates and majorly allows the body to modify its metabolism without being hungry. This regime is distinguished by the appearance of bodies called "ketones" in blood and urine. The liver produces ketones from fat whenever the body has fasted for more than one day or has absorbed sufficient calories from fat without being accompanied by fat. Among the ketones are acetoacetic acid, acetone (which is removed by exhaling and which produces a "fruity" smell when a person is suddenly in strong ketosis), and beta-hydroxybutyric acid. Chemically speaking, the latter is not a ketone, but physiologically it is assimilated to ketones because it appears wherever there is a production of acetoacetic acid.

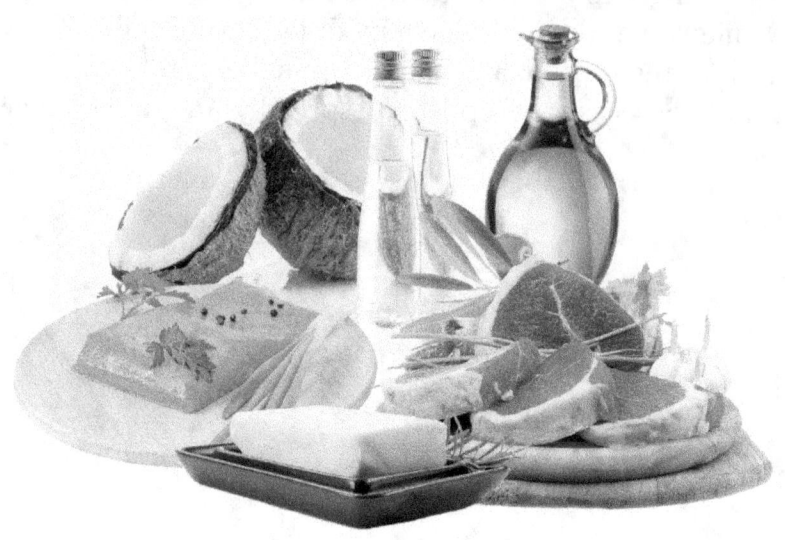

Principles behind the Ketogenic diet

Normally, the brain depends on a significant amount of glucose that emanates from the body converting the carbohydrates into the chemical. However, in some nutritional circumstances, the levels of carbohydrates in the diet are insufficient leading to the conversion of fat in the liver into fatty acids and chemical substances known as ketones. The fatty acids act as supplements for the body and brains' insufficient glucose levels. However, the results of the body turning to fats for energy conversion results in elevated levels of ketones in the blood, a conditions known as ketosis. Medical professionals realized that these elevated ketones seem to significantly influence the occurrence of epileptic seizures especially in younger individuals and children resulting in its use as an alternative form of medicine for these hard-to-treat conditions.

Permitted and avoidable foods:

Food allowed:

Fish, seafood, meat, poultry, eggs, butter, vegetable oil, vinegar, juice of lemon, olives, avocado, low-carbohydrate vegetables such as leafy green vegetables (spinach, lettuce all types, endive, cabbage kale, chard), cheese farms (maximum 100 g per day).

Foods allowed in moderation:

Dairy products such as milk (preferred whole milk 3.25%), the Mediterranean yogurts likely to 7-8% fat, more vegetables rich in carbohydrates (avoid carrots, beets, corn, parsnips, apple Earth, sweet potato, spaghetti squash, and green peas), wine, strong alcohol, coffee without sugar.

Foods to avoid:

- ✓ sugar,
- ✓ sugary products,
- ✓ grain products (breakfast cereals, bread, pasta, rice, couscous, quinoa, oatmeal, barley, buckwheat, crackers, muffins, pancakes, tortillas, pita, bagels, granola bar, And any other product made from flour such as pastries, donuts, biscuits, sweets),
- ✓ legumes,
- ✓ fruit (except berries which in some cases are allowed), soft cheeses (cottage, ricotta),
- ✓ Fresh cheese,
- ✓ rice-based and soy-based cheeses
- ✓ soft drinks, frozen desserts (frozen cream and yogurt), chocolate, white sugar, brown sugar, honey, maple syrup, Molasses, jams, fruit and vegetable juices, cereal coffees, sweet sauces, flavored soy milk or beverages, fruit compotes and fruit salads with added sugar.

Taking a multivitamin and a fiber supplement is recommended. Besides, it is recommended to stay well hydrated throughout the day by drinking 2.5 to 3 liters of water per day.

Types of fat to be preferred

As a significant amount of fat is ingested every day, it is important to care about the kind of fat. It is recommended to limit consumption of omega-6 fatty acid, which in excess, have a pro-inflammatory effect. The primary sources of omega-6 are soybean oils, corn, safflower, grapeseed, sunflower, and wheat germ. It is, therefore, necessary to limit the consumption of salad dressings, vinaigrettes, and mayonnaises based on these oils.

The consumption of monounsaturated fats (olive oil, avocado, nuts) and saturated fats (cuts of fatty meat, dairy products rich in fat) is advisable. The use of coconut oil is also recommended because it contains fat that is quickly processed into ketones.

Ketogenic diet for weight loss

According to various studies, the ketogenic diet for weight loss is characterized by the maximum consumption of 50 g of carbs per day representing around 5% of the calories consumed in the day. A typical diet usually provides between 45 and 65% of our calories in the form of carbohydrates. The remainder is distributed between lipids and proteins. In the ketogenic diet, the calories ingested in the form of lipids can reach up to 75%, and the proteins occupy the remaining 20%.

How does the ketogenic diet necessitate weight loss?

Usually, the body draws in the carbohydrates consumed in the day to the energy needed for proper functioning of the body. In this diet, carbohydrates being extremely limited, the body begins to tap into its stores of carbohydrates stored in the muscles and liver called "glycogen" stores. As each gram of glycogen is bound to 3-4 g of water in the body, significant early weight loss in the ketogenic diet is actually a loss of water. When glycogen stores are depleted, the body begins to use lipids or fats to produce energy. When the body uses fat in the absence of carbohydrates, it produces waste products called ketones. Next, the ketone bodies begin to accumulate in the blood and their odor, similar to that of nail polish, becomes perceptible in the breath. This is the primary indicator that the body is in a "ketosis" state. It takes around 2 to 4 weeks before arriving at this condition. The state of "ketosis" can be checked by obtaining strips of urine analysis in pharmacy.

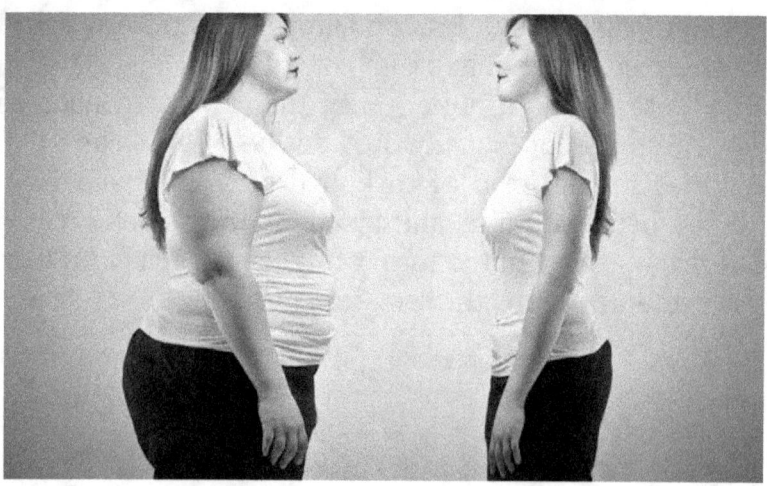

This state of "ketosis" causes a marked decrease in appetite, which contributes to reducing the amount of food consumed. This condition can also lead to nausea and fatigue. Although the scheme does not center on counting calories, those who follow the diet absorb fewer calories because they do not go hungry and this, therefore, leads to weight loss.

Tips to lose weight with the ketogenic diet

✓ You have to have available a composition table of food and culinary balance to quantify carbohydrates accurately.
✓ When tired, do not hesitate to take a vitamin supplementation.
✓ It is imperative to raise revenues ahead of plan. Cooking with the energy distribution imposed by the diet will otherwise quickly become a real headache.

In total, if the ketogenic diet can give a boost to losing 2 or 3 pounds quickly on a particular occasion, it cannot be followed long-term without health risks.

Example of ketogenic menu providing 1500 kcal

Breakfast

- ✓ Unsweetened coffee or tea (possibility of sweetener)
- ✓ 1 handle (30 g) of almonds, walnuts or hazelnuts
- ✓ 50 g of red fruits: strawberries, raspberries, blackcurrants, gooseberries

Lunch and dinner

- ✓ 50 g of raw vegetables (the equivalent of a small grated carrot), vinaigrette with 1 tablespoon of walnut or rapeseed oil
- ✓ 120 g of meat or fish or 2 eggs: cooking with 1 tablespoon of colza or olive oil
- ✓ 100 g vegetables + 2 teaspoons butter or 2 tablespoons whole cream
- ✓ To taste
- ✓ 60 g of cheese or 30 g of cheese + 1 ramekin of whole milk white cheese

KETOGENIC RECIPES

BREAKFAST

Keto Breakfast mocha

Ready in 5 minute

Servings: 4

Ingredients:
- ✓ One tablespoon of coconut oil
- ✓ One tablespoon of butter
- ✓ A spoonful of cocoa powder
- ✓ Sweetener to taste
- ✓ A big cup of very hot coffee
- ✓ One teaspoon of vanilla extract
- ✓ 2 tablespoons cream (optional)
- ✓

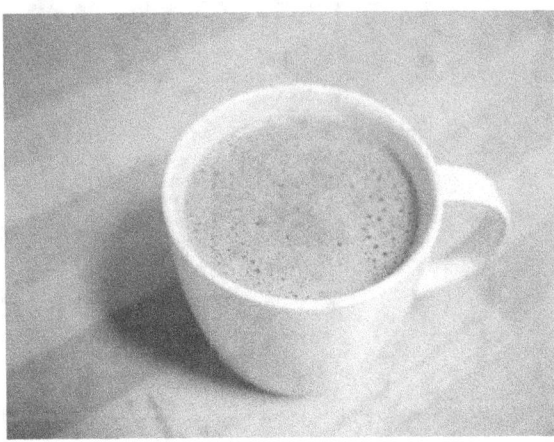

Preparation

1. Put all the ingredients in a heat resistant blender and blend.
2. Serve in a mug.

Prep Time: 10 Minutes

Cooking Time: 10 Minutes

Servings: 2

Ingredients

- ✓ 5 eggs
- ✓ Cilantro
- ✓ Salt
- ✓ 1 Avocado
- ✓ Pepper
- ✓ 2 Sweet potatoes
- ✓ Hot sauce
- ✓ Sausage
- ✓ Raw cheese

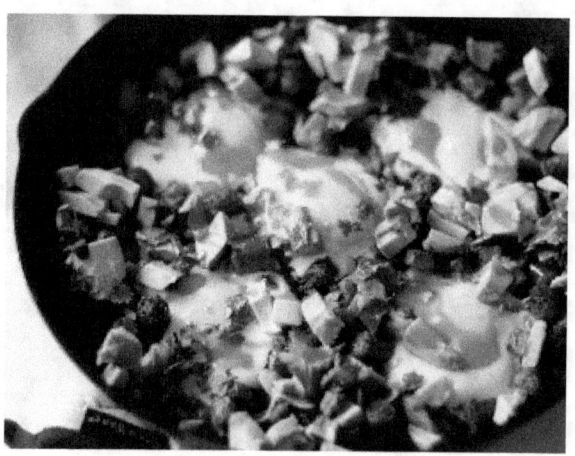

Preparation

1. Put a skillet over medium heat and add the sausage to crumble and brown.
2. Once brown, remove and add sweet potatoes to the sausage grease left in the skillet.
3. Once the potatoes get crispy, add the sausages back to the skillet.
4. Create wells in the food mixture in the skillet and crack the eggs into them.
5. Heat for 5-10 minutes and remove the skillet from the heat.
6. Douse the food with avocado and cilantro and serve.

Prep Time: 15 Minutes

Cooking Time: 30 Minutes

Servings: 3

Ingredients

- ✓ 100g fat cheese
- ✓ 12 slices of organic bacon
- ✓ 6 eggs, hard-cooked
- ✓ ¼ tsp. of dried organic thyme

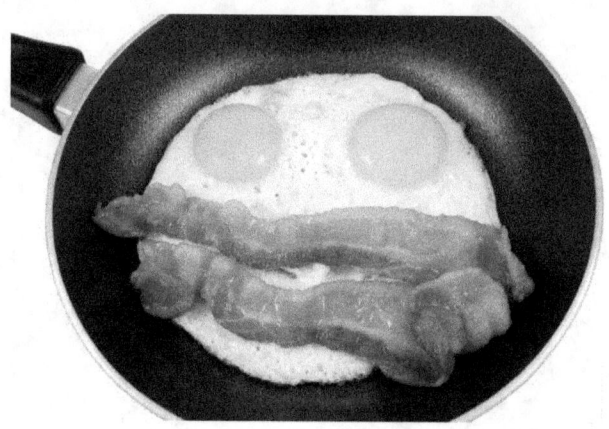

Preparation

1. Mix thyme and cream cheese in a bowl using a spoon and then cover and put aside.
2. Peel the eggs and cut them into halves.
3. Fill six halves with cream cheese and use the other halves to cover them.
4. Cut the bacon into slices and use them to cover the eggs.
5. Place the wrapped eggs in a ceramic baking dish in an oven and bake for 30 minutes.
6. Remove the food from the oven and serve.

<u>Ready in 30 minute</u>

<u>Servings: 15</u>

Ingredients
- ✓ 1 cup natural peanut butter
- ✓ 1 egg
- ✓ 1 cup sugar substitute
- ✓ 1 teaspoon vanilla
- ✓ Sea salt
- ✓ Honey

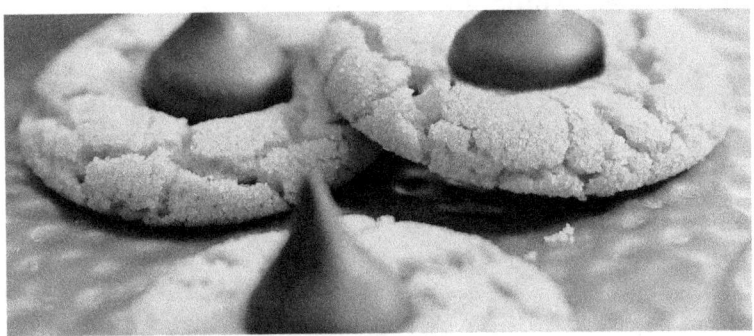

Preparation
1. Position 1 oven rack in upper 1/3 of oven and place a second rack in the lower 1/3 part of the oven. Heat oven to 350 degrees F.
2. In a medium-sized mixing bowl, combine peanut butter, egg, sugar substitute, and vanilla. Stir until all is well combined.
3. Drop by a tablespoon onto an ungreased cookie sheet, keeping 1 inch apart from each other. Flatten with a fork in a crisscross design and sprinkle with sea salt.
4. Bake in oven for 5 minutes on upper rack. Move to lower rack for another 5 minutes. Continue baking until golden brown along the edges. Remove and transfer to waxed paper.
5. Drizzle with a little warmed honey.

Prep Time: 10 Minutes

Cooking Time: 10 Minutes

Servings: 2

Ingredients

- ✓ 2 eggs
- ✓ ½ teaspoon of cinnamon
- ✓ Cream cheese
- ✓ 1 teaspoon of granulated sugar substitute

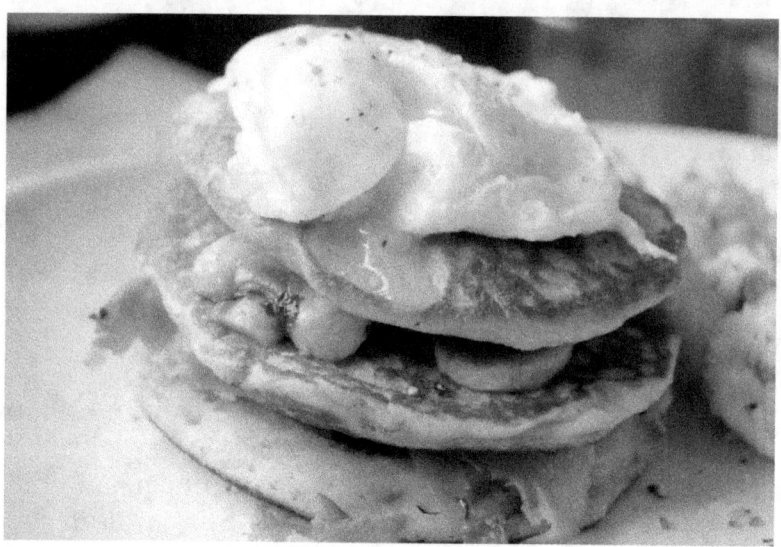

Preparation

1. Place all the ingredients in a blender and blend until smooth.
2. Pour the batter on a cooking pan and cook until brown then flip the other side.
3. Remove and serve with fresh berries and sugar free syrup.

Prep Time: 12 hours 10 minutes

Servings: 1

Ingredients

- ✓ ½ tablespoon of honey
- ✓ 1 cup of coconut milk
- ✓ ¼ cup of chia seeds
- ✓ Nuts

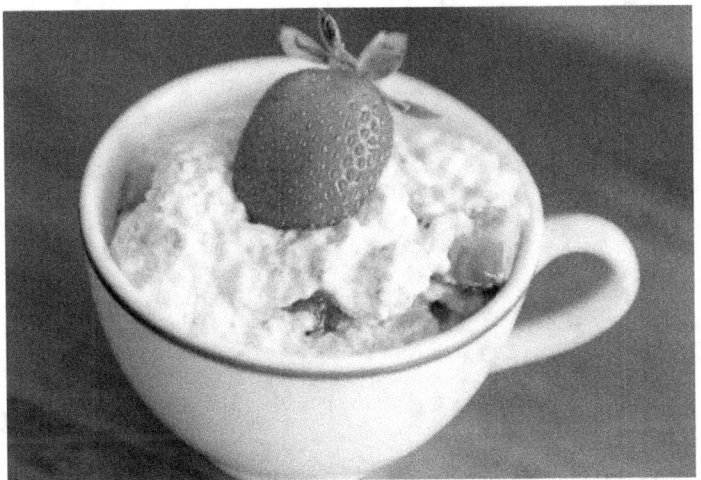

Preparation

1. Mix honey, coconut milk and chia seeds in a bowl and put in a refrigerator for at least 6 hours.
2. Remove it from the fridge, add nuts or fresh fruit, and enjoy your breakfast.

Prep Time: 10 Minutes

Cooking Time: 10 Minutes

Servings: 2

Ingredients

- ✓ 6 eggs
- ✓ Salt to taste
- ✓ 1 green onion
- ✓ 1 breakfast sausage, pound

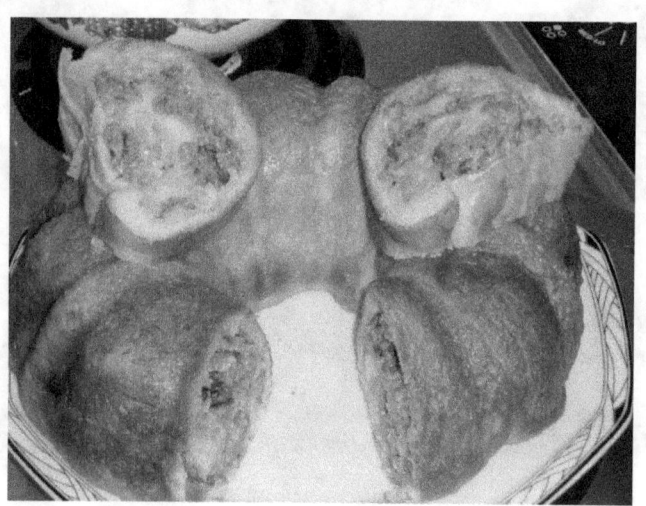

Preparation

1. Heat the oven to 350° F.
2. Divide the sausage into different portions and place each on a ramekin.
3. Use a spoon to push the sausage such that a crust is created.
4. Crack the eggs into the crusts created in the sausages.
5. Add green onion and salt.
6. Bake for 30 minutes in the oven.
7. Remove and enjoy.

Prep Time: 10 Minutes

Cooking Time: 15 Minutes

Servings: 2

Ingredients

- ✓ Spinach
- ✓ Coconut oil
- ✓ Spices-salt and pepper
- ✓ Frozen mix of cauliflower, broccoli, carrots and green beans
- ✓ 2 eggs

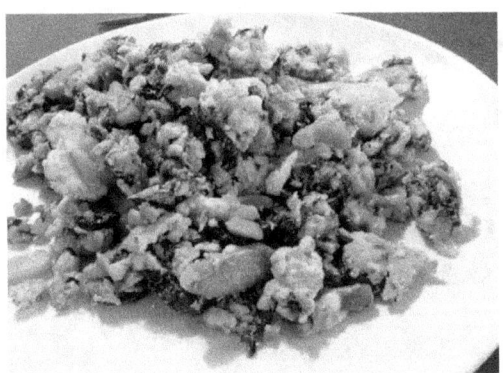

Preparation

1. Put a frying pan on moderate heat and add coconut oil.
2. Add the frozen mix of vegetables and let it thaw for at least 5 minutes.
3. Add the eggs.
4. Add salt and pepper to taste.
5. Add spinach then stir for at least 10 minutes.
6. Serve and enjoy.

<u>Ready in 1minute</u>

<u>Servings: 2</u>

Ingredients
- ✓ Two passion fruits
- ✓ 1 mango
- ✓ One egg white, beaten until stiff peaks have formed

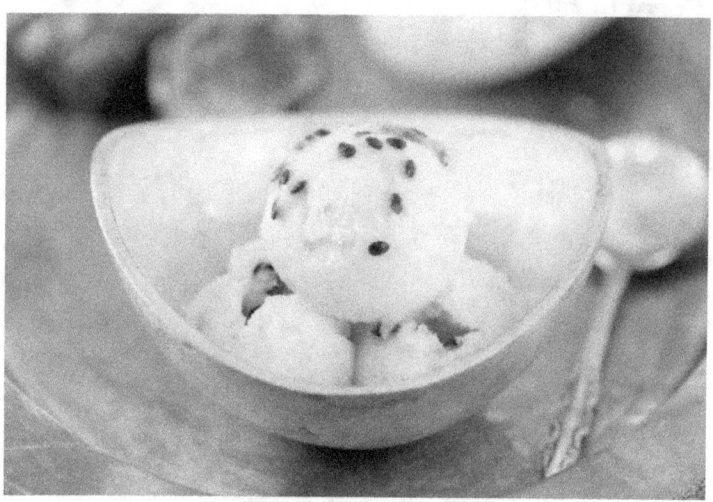

Method:

1. In a bowl, beat the egg whites till you have stiff peaks. Blend the mango and passion fruit together till you have a creamy texture.
2. Fold the egg whites into the mango mixture. Pour it into a freezer proof container and freeze for 6 hours or until it has set. While serving cut into slices and top it with mango or passion fruit slices.

2 servings

Ingredients
- ✓ 1 shot espresso
- ✓ One scoop vanilla protein powder
- ✓ Five ice cubes
- ✓ ¼ cup Greek yogurt
- ✓ Pinch cinnamon
- ✓ Pinch Stevia

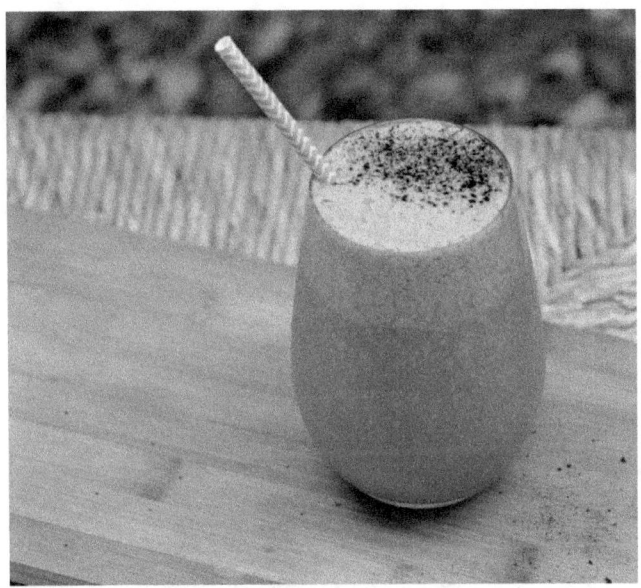

Preparation
1. Mix everything in a blender.
2. Enjoy

LUNCH

<u>Ready in 35 minute</u>

<u>Servings: 3</u>

Ingredients
- ✓ 8 eggs
- ✓ 1 bowl of fresh cream
- ✓ 1 bowl of grated cheese
- ✓ Salt and pepper
- ✓ 1 clove of garlic, minced

Filling:
- ✓ 100 gr fried mushrooms
- ✓ 100 or 100 gr shrimp cooked ground meat and 100 grams of peppers, or cooked chicken breast and 100 gr feta.

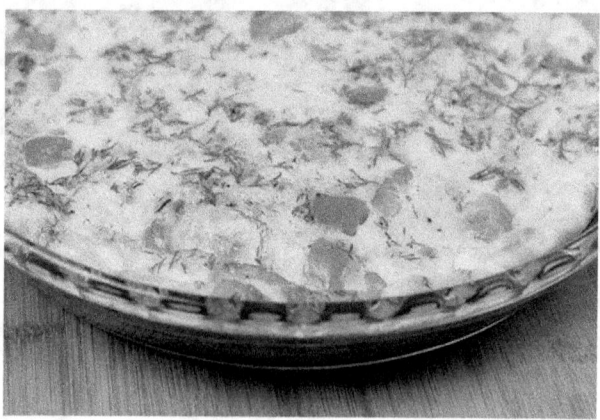

Preparation
1. Beat eggs with cream, chopped clove of garlic, salt and pepper in a bowl.
2. Place the toppings of your choice into muffin molds and pour over eggs preparedness.
3. Bake at 180 degrees for 15 minutes.

Prep Time: 10 Minutes

Servings: 3

Ingredients

- ✓ 1 green onion, minced
- ✓ 1 celery ribs, minced
- ✓ 5 ounces of chicken breast meat
- ✓ ¼ teaspoon of garlic
- ✓ 1 boiled egg, chopped
- ✓ 1 teaspoon of mustard
- ✓ Salt
- ✓ Pepper
- ✓ 1/3 cup of mayonnaise
- ✓ 2 tablespoons of parsley

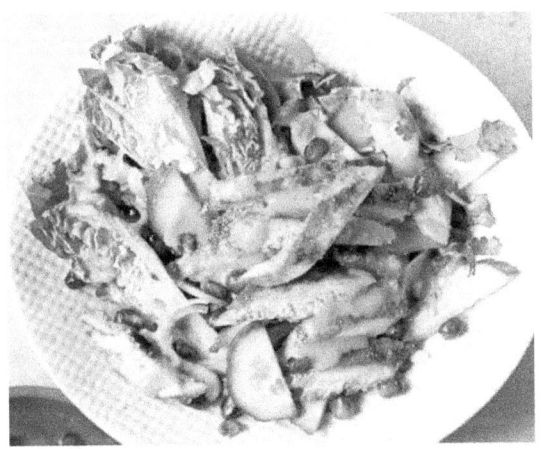

Preparation

1. Put celery, parsley and onions in a food processor bowl.
2. Pulse until they become fine then transfer to a mixing bowl.
3. Add chicken and pulse.
4. Grate the egg and add to the mixing bowl.
5. Add mustard and mix well using a spoon.
6. Season to taste with salt and pepper and keep in refrigerator while inside an airtight container for a week.
7. Serve and enjoy.

<u>Ready in 1 Hour 10 minute</u>

<u>Servings: 6</u>

Ingredients
- ✓ 750 grams of minced meat with fat
- ✓ 1 medium onion
- ✓ 3 green peppers
- ✓ 3 tablespoons tomato paste
- ✓ 1 tomato, diced
- ✓ 1 tablespoon Mexican seasoning
- ✓ 2 garlic clove
- ✓ 5 cl olive oil
- ✓ Salt and pepper

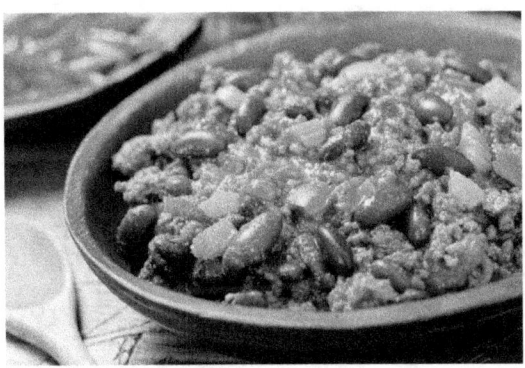

Preparation
1. Cut the onion and diced peppers, crush the garlic and fry in a pan with half of the olive oil
2. Fry the minced meat, salt and pepper in a pan.
3. Add the chopped tomatoes and diced tomato paste to the pot with the Mexican seasoning, the rest of the olive oil and cooked ground meat.
4. Cook everything over very low heat for one hour.

Fennel Walnut Chicken Salad

<u>Prep Time: 20 Minutes</u>

<u>Servings: 6</u>

Ingredients

- ✓ 3 boneless chicken breasts
- ✓ 2 cloves of garlic
- ✓ ¼ teaspoon of cayenne
- ✓ 2 tablespoons of fennel fronds, chopped
- ✓ 2 tablespoons of lemon juice, freshly squeezed
- ✓ 2 tablespoons of walnut oil
- ✓ ¼ cup of mayonnaise
- ✓ ¼ cup of toasted walnuts
- ✓ 2 cups of fresh fennel

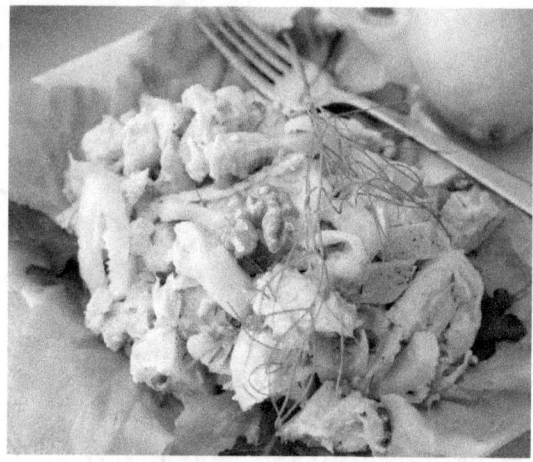

Preparation

1. Toss fennel, walnut and cooked chicken in a large bowl.
2. Whisk mayonnaise, lemon juice, walnut oil, garlic, fennel fronds, and cayenne in another bowl.
3. Pour the dressing over the mixture of chicken.
4. Toss and season with pepper and salt.
5. Put the salad in a refrigerator for at least 6 hours.
6. Serve and enjoy your meal.

Prep Time: 10 Minutes

Servings: 2

Ingredients

- ✓ 1 large avocado
- ✓ 1 onion
- ✓ ¼ tablespoon salt
- ✓ ¼ teaspoon of turmeric powder
- ✓ 1 tablespoon of lemon juice, fresh
- ✓ 1 tin of sardines
- ✓ 1 tablespoon of mayonnaise

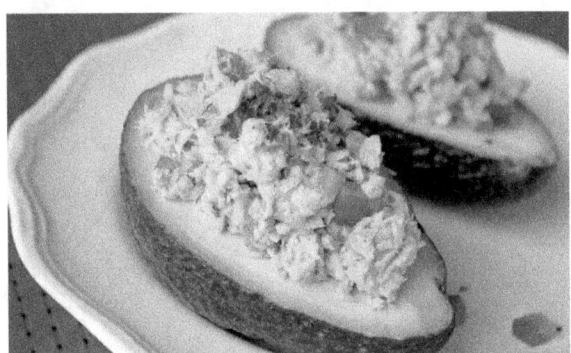

Preparation

1. Cut the avocado into half and remove the seed.
2. Drain the sardines and break them into pieces then place in a bowl.
3. Scoop the middle part of the avocado and place in a small bowl leaving only an inch of the flesh.
4. Add the sliced onions and turmeric powder to the bowl containing sardines.
5. Add mayonnaise to the bowl with sardines and mix well.
6. Mix the contents of the two bowls and squeeze in lemon juice then season with salt.
7. Scoop the mixture into the two halves of avocado and enjoy.

Fried chicken with coconut flour

<u>Ready in 25 minute</u>

<u>Servings: 6</u>

Ingredients
- 2 kg of chicken thighs (up and pestle)
- Salt pepper
- Garlic powder or two garlic cloves mashed
- 1 tablespoon paprika
- 100 grams of coconut flour
- Oil for frying

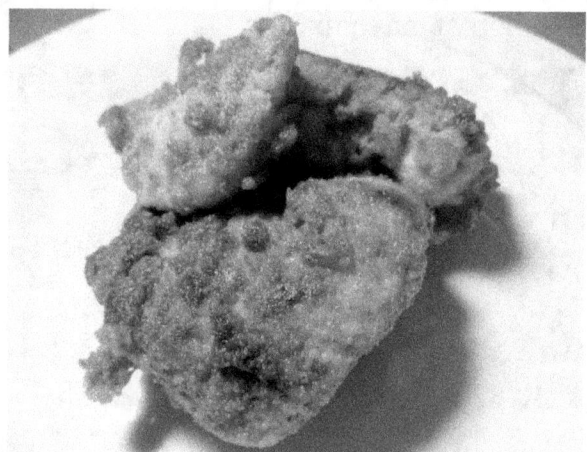

Preparation
- ✓ Marinade: In a large bowl, combine the chicken, salt, pepper, garlic and paprika. Mix well with your hands and make sure the spices cover the entire surface of the chicken. Marinate for at least two hours. It is better to marinate the night before.
- ✓ Breading the chicken marinated in coconut flour, heat oil in a deep fryer or saucepan to 190 °. Fry chicken, being careful not to put too much at once so that the chicken becomes crispy. Cook 8 minutes on each side until chicken pieces are golden.
- ✓ Rune thigh cut in two to make sure the meat is not pink in the interior.

Ready in 45 minute

Servings: 6

Ingredients
- ✓ 150 grams of smoked salmon
- ✓ A large bowl of cooked spinach (revenues in butter)
- ✓ 100 grams of cheese cream cheese with garlic and herbs
- ✓ A handful of grated cheese

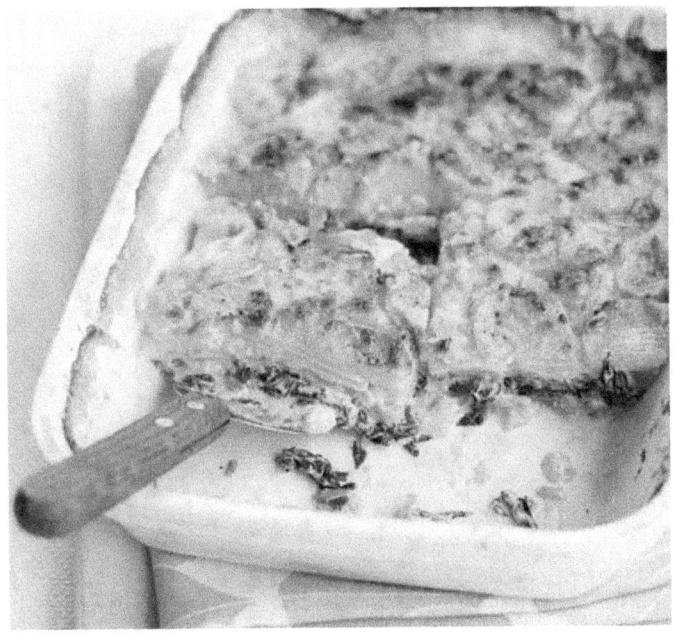

Preparation
1. Mix the spinach with cream cheese, gently add the smoked salmon. Put in a baking dish and sprinkle with grated cheese.
2. Put in a hot oven.

Prep time 3mins. Cooking time 25min. 1 portion.

Ingredients
- ✓ 2 eggs
- ✓ A small bowl of tomato sauce
- ✓ 500 grams of minced meat
- ✓ Half a pepper cut into washer
- ✓ Half onion cut into thin slices
- ✓ 2 tablespoons grated Parmesan cheese
- ✓ 150 grams of grated cheese
- ✓ Salt and pepper
- ✓ Tabasco

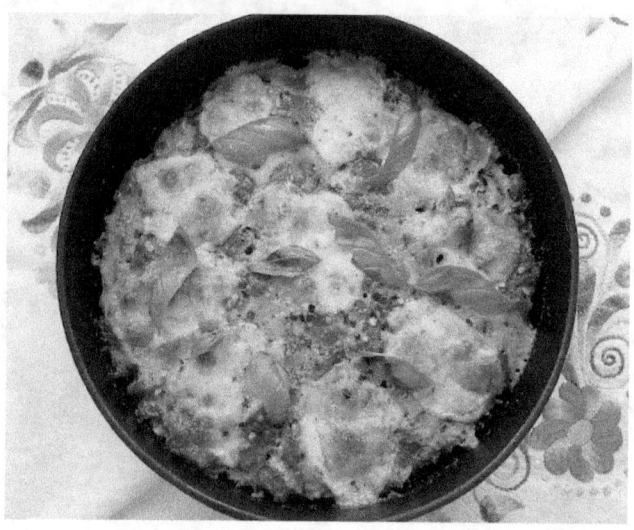

Preparation
1. Add salt and pepper to the chopped meat, add two beaten eggs, 2 tablespoons grated Parmesan and shape as a pizza dough in a baking dish.
2. Garnish with tomato sauce, peppers, onions, a few drops of Tabasco sauce and grated cheese.
3. Bake for 20 minutes at 200 degrees. Serve with a salad.

<u>Ready in 35 minute</u>

<u>Servings: 3</u>

Ingredients:
- ✓ 1 kg of ' bone beef or a chicken carcass
- ✓ A sprig of thyme
- ✓ 2 bay leaves
- ✓ A beautiful celery
- ✓ A small bunch of parsley
- ✓ 5 peppercorns (or pepper)
- ✓ 2 cloves of garlic
- ✓ 1 carrot cut into thick trogons
- ✓ Half of a medium onion
- ✓ 1 leek cut into thick sections
- ✓ A teaspoon salt
- ✓ 4 tbsps. cider vinegar
- ✓ 2 tablespoons chopped parsley

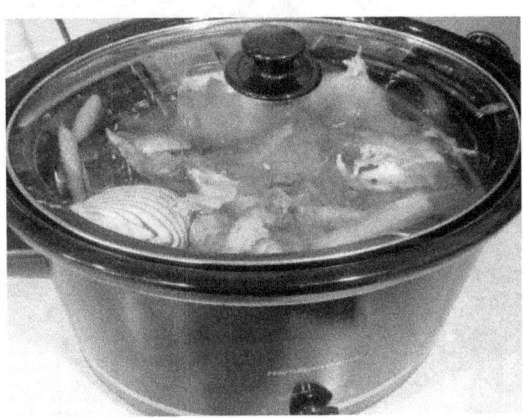

Preparation
1. In a Dutch oven or casserole, put the oil to heat; add the bones, pods of garlic, peppercorns, salt and vegetables. Make a bouquet garni with thyme, bay leaf, parsley and celery, put in the pan, cover with water and cook over low heat for half past one.
2. Pass the bones and vegetables in a colander to keep only the liquid.
3. Sprinkle with chopped parsley before serving.

Ready in 25 minutes

Servings: 6

Ingredients
- ✓ 1 large bunch of spinach
- ✓ 1 bunch chopped parsley and coriander
- ✓ 5 chopped cloves of garlic
- ✓ 10 cl of oil olive
- ✓ 1/2 lemon
- ✓ 1 c. tablespoon paprika
- ✓ 1/2 c. Coffee pepper
- ✓ 1 c. salt coffee
- ✓ 100g of red olives

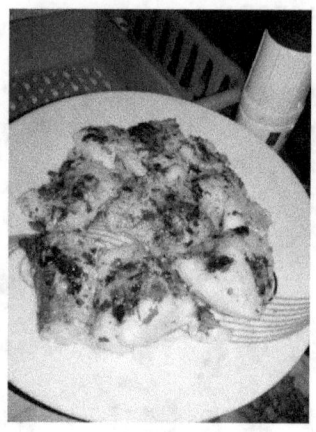

Preparation
1. In a large wok or hot frying pan, add oil, crushed garlic cloves, chopped parsley and coriander, spices and salt, cook 5 minutes over low heat and add the chopped spinach coarsely.
2. Simmer preparation for 10 minutes, stirring constantly.
3. Before serving, garnish with olives red spinach and thin strips of candied lemon.

Ready in 15 minutes

Servings:2

Ingredients
- ✓ 1 lb. mushrooms
- ✓ ½ cup chicken broth
- ✓ 8 ounces Boursin cheese
- ✓ Paprika to garnish

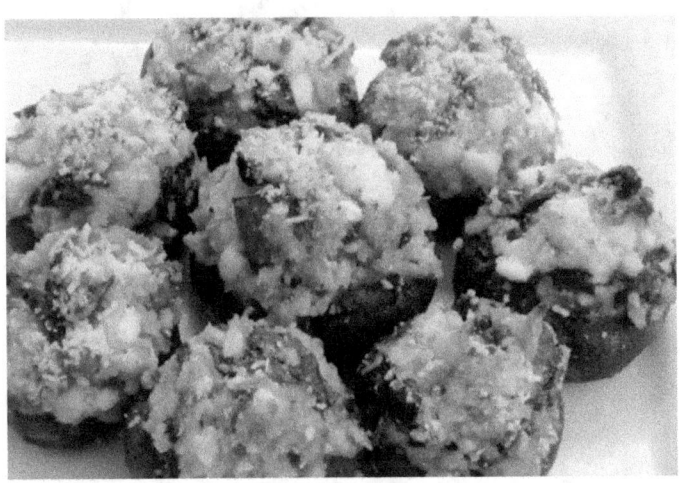

Instructions
1. Preheat the oven to 350 degrees F. Remove the stems from the mushrooms, and reserve them for another use.
2. Fill all the mushrooms with Boursin, and place them in a baking pan.
3. Pour some chicken broth around the mushrooms to fill the bottom of the pan.
4. Spread lightly with paprika.
5. Bake for 30 to 40 minutes and serve hot.

Ready after 50 minutes,

6 servings

Ingredients

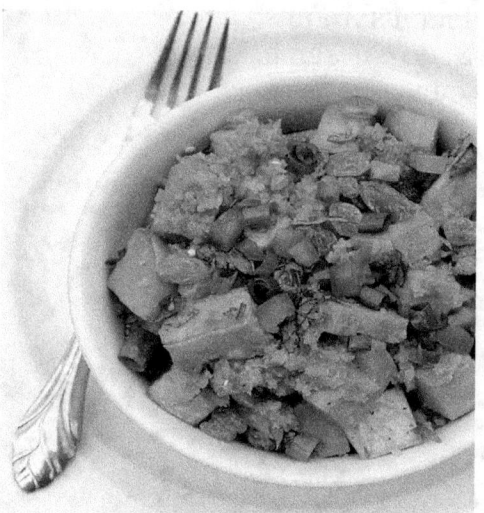

- ½ cup of extra virgin olive oil
- ¼ cup red wine vinegar
- 2 teaspoons cumin (ground)
- ½ cup sliced scallion
- 2 fresh minced chilies
- 4 large sweet potatoes
- Freshly ground pepper and salt
- ¼ cup raisins (not a must)
- 1 cored, seeded, and medium sized quartered red bell pepper
- 1 tablespoon grated orange zest
- ½ cup minced fresh mint leaves

Preparation

1. Get your oven ready by preheating it to 400 degrees F
2. Cut your sweet potatoes to bite size pieces after peeling them. Take two tablespoons of the oil and while placing the potatoes on a baking sheet, sprinkle them with the oil and coat them by tossing.
3. Using your salt and pepper, sprinkle the potatoes and get them roasted with occasional turning until they are tender inside and brown on the outside. This could take around thirty minutes.
4. Stop cooking and place them on a pan.
5. Dress the potatoes as they cook and add the remaining oil blender, about 6 tablespoons. Add also bell pepper, zest, cumin and vinegar then use little pepper and salt to sprinkle the potatoes. Smooth them by pureeing.
6. Since you have mint, scallion, raisins, and chilies, use them to toss the warm potatoes. Add the dressing (as much as required) and toss until well coated. Serve immediately.

Red pepper and lentil bake

Ready after 1 hour 30 minutes

4 servings

Ingredients

- 1 large onion, peeled and finely chopped
- 1/2 cup lentil
- 4 red bell peppers, deseeded and chopped
- 2 teaspoons dried basil
- 1 ounce shredded cheddar cheese
- 14 ounces canned and chopped tomatoes
- 1/3 ounce shredded parmesan cheese
- 2 1/2 cups low-sodium, organic vegetable broth
- Salt and pepper to taste
- 1/4 cup white wine
- 1 teaspoon olive oil
- 1 large cooking apple such as Granny Smith or McIntosh, peeled, cored, and chopped
- 1 garlic clove, peeled and finely chopped

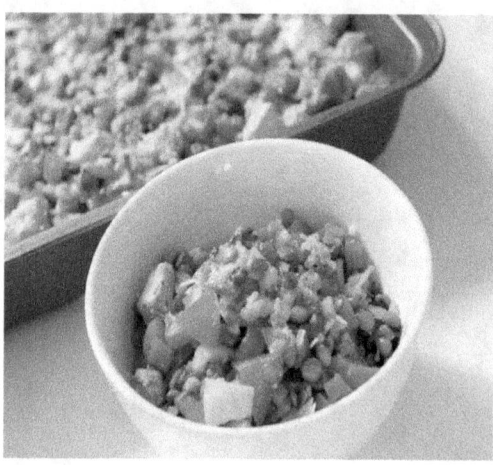

Preparation
1. Prepare the oven by preheating it to 350 degrees.
2. Put the olive oil in a saucepan and heat it. Add garlic and onion and fry them until the onions are observed to be translucent.
3. Take your lentils, add them and stir then add vegetable stock bringing it to boil. Reduce the heat and cook for about 30 minutes.
4. Add the canned tomatoes, white wine, peppers, apple, and basil then mix them very well.
5. Place the mixture in an oven proof 8 by 14 baking dish sprinkling cheese on top. Cook for 35 minutes.
6. It is best when immediately served.

Ready after 1 hour

6 servings

Ingredients
- 3 cups chopped tomatoes
- 1 pound diced sweet potatoes
- 1/4 teaspoon salt
- 1 tablespoon olive oil
- 2 1/2 teaspoons ground cumin
- 1 diced red pepper
- Salt and pepper, to taste
- 1/2 teaspoon cayenne pepper
- 4 15-ounces can black beans
- hole-wheat tortilla wraps
- 1 cup frozen corn

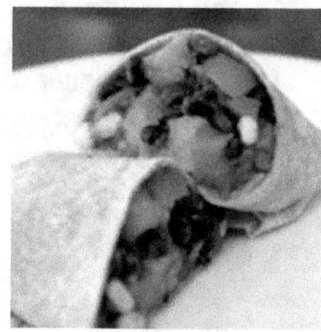

Preparation
1. Get your oven ready by preheating it to 400 degrees.
2. Place your sweet potatoes in a pan and toss them with 1/4 teaspoon salt, ¼ teaspoon cumin, and olive oil then roast them for 30 minutes. Cook them until they turn brown and are soft.
3. Keep roasting and add black beans, red pepper, tomatoes, corn, cumin and cayenne to a large pot and cook for 20 minutes.
4. Get a plate wrapped then for 20 seconds, microwave it until it becomes warm and softens. Into the center of the tortilla, spoon out ¼ of the mixture of tomato and beans.
5. Add a quarter of the roasted potatoes. Fold all sides of the wrap. Now place on a plate and eat.

DINNER

<u>Ready in 35 minutes</u>

<u>Servings: 5</u>

Ingredients
- ✓ 2 small eggplants
- ✓ 200 g sausage meat
- ✓ 20 tbsp. to s. olive oil
- ✓ 6 tbsp. to s. tomato paste
- ✓ 1 tsp. c. paprika
- ✓ 2 cloves garlic
- ✓ 4 basil leaves
- ✓ 2 tbsp. to s. heavy cream
- ✓ 2 tbsp. to s. of grated pecorino
- ✓ 2 balls of mozzarella
- ✓ Sea salt

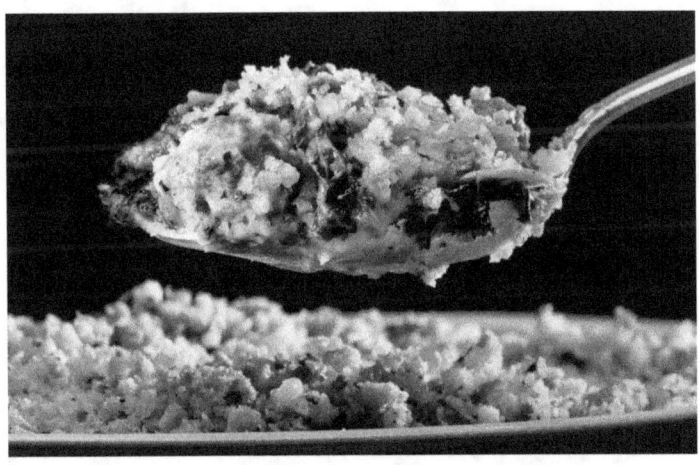

Preparation
1. Wash and cut the eggplant into thin slices. Add salt and leave in a colander disgorge. Brown the sausage meat in an oiled pan, set aside. In the same skillet, brown the eggplant and let them cook with olive oil.
2. Peel and slice the garlic. Chop the basil. Mix tomato paste with chili, garlic, basil and a little water. Slice the mozzarella.
3. Preheat oven to 365F. In a baking dish, arrange a layer of eggplant.
4. Cover succession of tomato sauce, cream, sausage and mozzarella. Repeat to superimpose all these ingredients. Finish with pecorino. Brown in the oven for 20 min.

Ready in 30 minutes

Servings: 4

Ingredients
- ✓ 4 large tomatoes
- ✓ 1 clove garlic + 1 small onion diced
- ✓ 2 c. to s. olive oil
- ✓ 10 chopped basil leaves

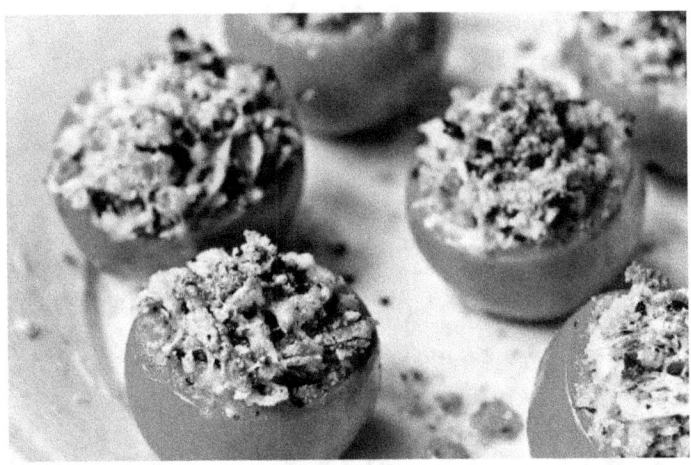

Preparation
1. Wash tomatoes and cut the upper part so as to detach a hat. Digging tomatoes and reserve the flesh. Rinse quinoa and cook in 2 times its volume of water. Once the water absorbed (about 15 minutes), cover and let stand.
2. Fry garlic and onion in olive oil for 3 minutes. Add the tomato flesh and basil. Salt and pepper.
3. Mix well and stuff the tomatoes.

<u>Ready in 55 minutes</u>

<u>Servings: 5</u>

Ingredients
- ✓ 1 kg of Canada gray apples
- ✓ 1/2 lemon
- ✓ 125 g of buckwheat flour
- ✓ 125g ground almonds
- ✓ 100g margarine with Omega-3
- ✓ 100 g sugar
- ✓ 1 c. c. ground cinnamon
- ✓ Olive oil

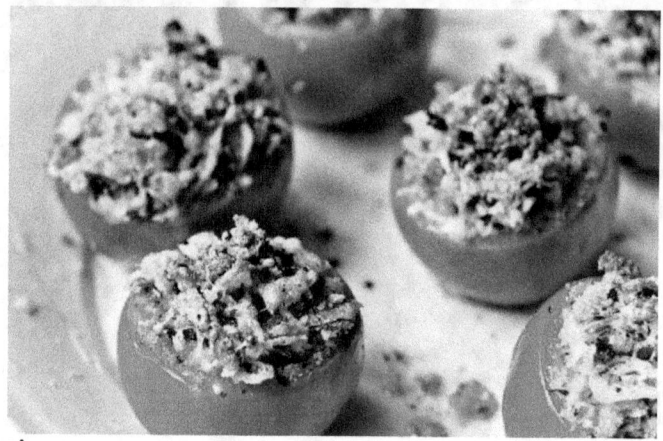

Preparation
1. Preheat oven to 376 F. Oil a baking dish (preferably Pyrex). Peel and cut apples into thin slices. Put them in the dish and sprinkle with lemon juice.
2. Bake for 10 to 15 minutes (possibly stir halfway through cooking). Meanwhile, put buckwheat flour, ground almonds, sugar and margarine in a bowl. Add cinnamon.
3. Mix for coarse sand. Remove the dish from the oven, mix some apples and crumble over the pastry. Bake 10 minutes, then turn off and let the dish in the oven for another 10 minutes. Serve warm.

Ready in 45 minutes

Servings: 5

Ingredients
- ✓ 1 red cabbage
- ✓ 2 apple tart flesh
- ✓ 200 g of natural chestnut
- ✓ 1 onion
- ✓ 1 c. to s. olive oil
- ✓ Thyme
- ✓ 5 bay leaves
- ✓ Herb salt

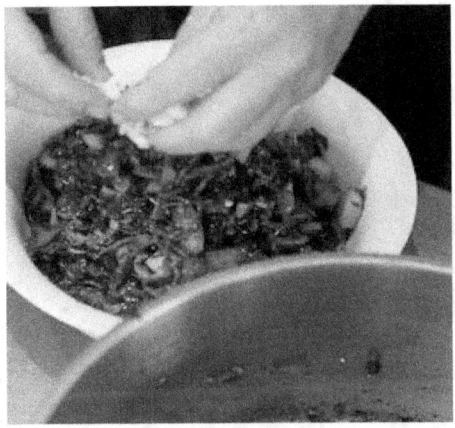

Preparation
1. Remove the hard core cabbage then cut it into thin strips.
2. Add the bay leaves, cover the cabbage strips sprinkled with thyme and some salt with herbs. Bake about 10 minutes.
3. Meanwhile, in a saucepan, melt over very low heat, without browning, onion finely chopped in olive oil and remaining thyme.
4. Add the cabbage and chestnuts, mix then put over the apples cut into thick slices. When the potatoes are cooked, serve immediately.

Ready in 30 minutes

Servings: 4

Ingredients

- ✓ 500 ml of water
- ✓ 40 g of chopped tomatoes
- ✓ 35 g of raw almonds or cashews (or sunflower seeds)
- ✓ 1/4 c. garlic powder
- ✓ 1/2 c. onion powder
- ✓ salt
- ✓ 1/2 c. lemon juice
- ✓ 2 c. arrowroot
- ✓ 25g flaked yeast

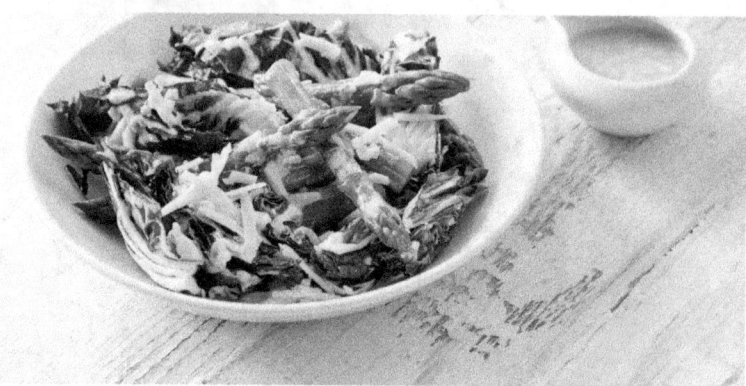

Preparation

1. Mix all ingredients in a blender until the mixture obtained is smooth. Then put the mixture in a saucepan and cook over low heat stirring constantly until it thickens.

Ready in 1 hour 10 minutes

Servings: 5

Ingredients
- ✓ 500g butternut squash
- ✓ 2 fennel bulbs
- ✓ 2 onions
- ✓ ½ glass 25cl vegetable broth
- ✓ Thyme, herb salt
- ✓ 2 pinches of grated nutmeg
- ✓ 2 large garlic cloves
- ✓ 125 g of rice flour
- ✓ 50 g of finely ground nuts
- ✓ Olive oil

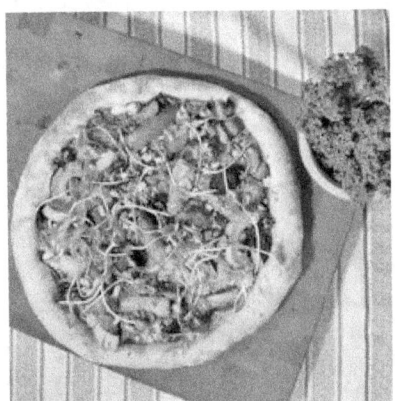

Preparation
1. Peel and cut squash into large "fries" very thick, thinly slice the fennel and onions.
2. Pour the vegetable stock into the bottom of a glass baking dish and garnish the dish by inserting rows of squash, onion and fennel.
3. Tighten rows. Drizzle lightly with olive oil. Prepare the crumble topping by mixing in a bowl the flour and nuts which added little by little olive oil until you notice the consistency of lumpy dough that kneads your fingertips.
4. Spread nutmeg, chopped garlic cloves and crumble over the vegetables. Bake at 110 ° C and cook until vegetables are melting.

<u>Ready in 1 hour 20 minutes</u>

<u>Servings: 5</u>

Ingredients

- ✓ 250g fillet of venison
- ✓ 100g mushrooms
- ✓ 25 g walnuts / pine nuts
- ✓ Chopped parsley
- ✓ ½ onion
- ✓ 1 garlic clove
- ✓ 300 g shallots
- ✓ 200 ml port
- ✓ Cinnamon
- ✓ 300 ml red wine
- ✓ 100 g of honey
- ✓ Olive oil
- ✓ Salt
- ✓ pepper

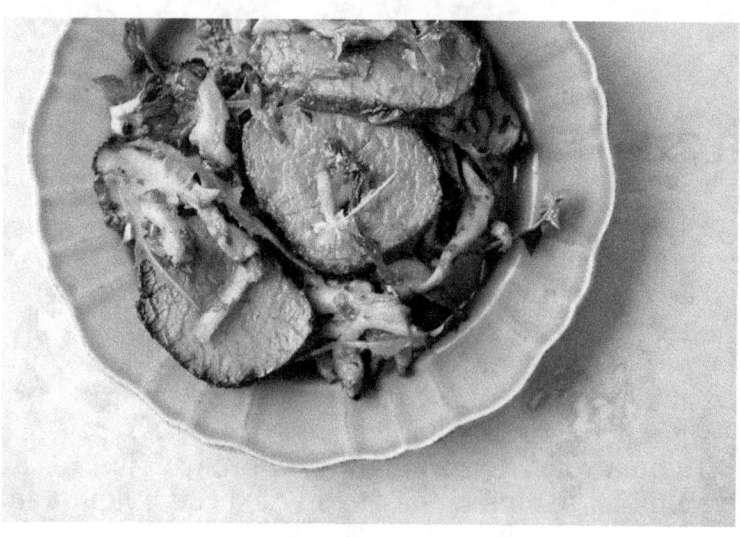

Preparation

1. Make confit slowly over low heat the shallots and garlic in wine mixture, port, honey, cinnamon and seasoning for 1 hour.

2. Place the piece of meat in the marinade once the cooled mixture. Fry the mushrooms in olive oil with chopped onion, walnuts and pine nuts and season. Roast meat piece at 200 ° C for 8 minutes.

3. Heat garlic and shallots and use the wine to water the piece of meat after cooking and make a sauce.

4. Serve the dish by arranging around the piece of meat the mixture of mushrooms, shallots, garlic, parsley, and drizzle with sauce just before serving.

<u>Ready in 35 minutes</u>

<u>Servings: 5</u>

Ingredients
- ✓ A beautiful salmon fillet 400g
- ✓ 2 tablespoons mustard
- ✓ 2 tablespoons olive oil
- ✓ Juice of half a lemon
- ✓ 4 tablespoons chopped chives
- ✓ Salt and pepper

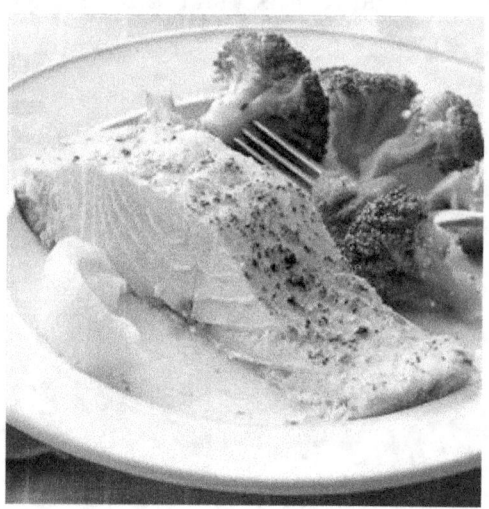

Preparation
1. Combine mustard, olive oil, lemon juice, 3 tablespoons chives cut, salt and pepper. Coat the salmon steak with this mixture and place in a baking dish.
2. Bake 15-20 minutes at 180 °. We need salmon remains soft. Serve with blanched vegetables income in olive oil, garlic and parsley.

Ready in 25 minutes

Servings: 3

Ingredients
- ✓ 300g turkey or ground chicken
- ✓ Emmenthal
- ✓ Salt
- ✓ Pepper
- ✓ Nutmeg
- ✓ ½ grated onion (2 tablespoons)
- ✓ 1 clove garlic, minced

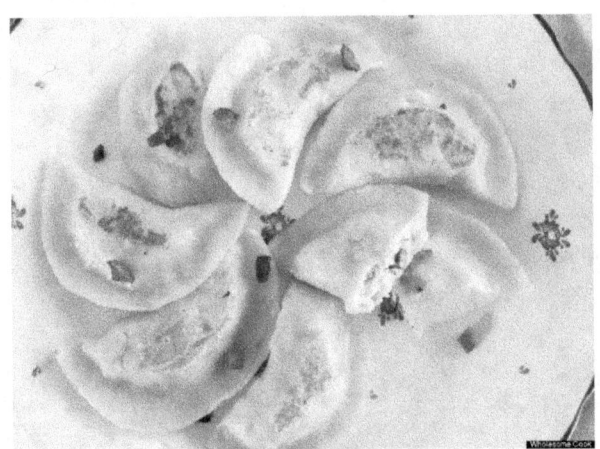

Preparation
1. Mix ground chicken with spices and onion and chopped garlic, make dumplings by putting Emmenthal center cubes. Put in a dish oiled oven.
2. Cook until the dumplings are golden.

Ready in 30 minutes

Servings: 5

Ingredients
- ✓ 400 g broccoli, washed and chopped
- ✓ 200 gr of zucchini cut into dice
- ✓ 1 leek
- ✓ 50g butter
- ✓ Salt pepper
- ✓ Cheese

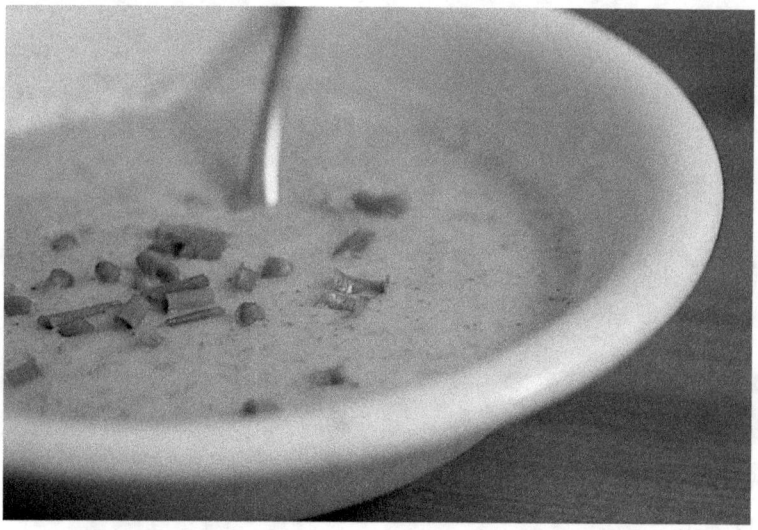

Preparation:
1. In a pan, put the butter to melt, add the leek cut and melt. Then add the chopped vegetables, mixing well.
2. Wet vegetables until almost cover and cook for twenty minutes.
3. Mix everything with cheese to make a soup, add salt and pepper.
4. serve

Ready in 35 minutes

Servings: 4

Ingredients
- ✓ 1 kg of lamb cut into the shoulder
- ✓ 1 chopped onion
- ✓ 1 large tomato, peeled, seeded and chopped
- ✓ 2 cloves garlic, minced
- ✓ 1 c. freshly ground black pepper
- ✓ 1 c. Coffee ginger
- ✓ 1 c. Coffee turmeric
- ✓ 4 cl oil
- ✓ 1 bunch coriander and parsley
- ✓ Salt
- ✓ Water
- ✓ For the vegetables:
- ✓ Oil for frying

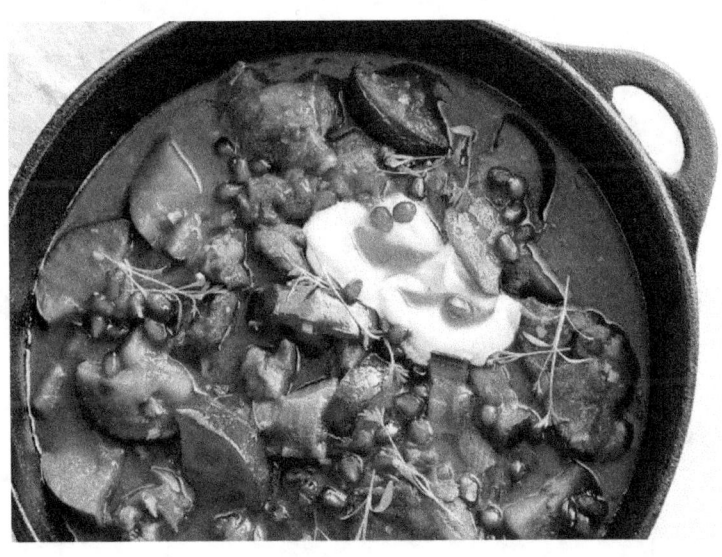

Preparation

1. In a pot over low heat, Place the pieces of meat and add onion, garlic, tomatoes, spices, salt and oil. Fry for about 10 minutes. Moisten up with water, cover the pot and bring to boil.
2. After boiling, add the bouquet of herbs and cook it all under cover and over low heat.
3. Wash the eggplant and detail in 1.5 cm thick slices.
4. Salt the eggplant slices and let drain for 10 minutes, rinse, squeeze between the palms and pat dry.
5. When the meat and chickpeas are cooked (fluxes) and the reduced sauce, remove the bouquet of coriander and parsley.
6. In a serving dish, prepare the meat, cover with sauce and garnish with fried eggplant.
7. Serve hot tagine.

Ready in 50 minutes

Servings: 6

Ingredients
- ✓ 500 grams of chicken Needles
- ✓ 50 grams of butter
- ✓ 100 cl of fresh cream
- ✓ 100 gram cheese
- ✓ 2 eggs
- ✓ A clove of garlic
- ✓ Salt
- ✓ Pepper

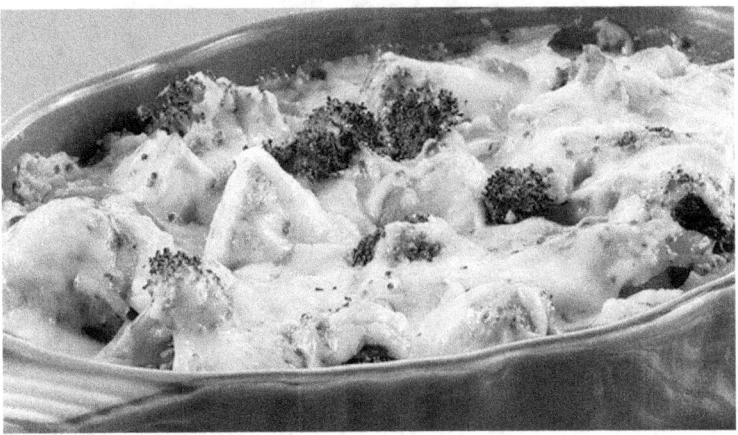

Preparation
1. Cook the broccoli in a pot of water for 10 minutes. It must remain firm.
2. Melt the butter in a pan, add the crushed garlic clove and salt and pepper chicken. Let brown.
3. Drain the broccoli and mix the chicken. Beat the eggs with the cream, salt and pepper. Put the broccoli and chicken in a baking dish, cover with the cream mixture and sprinkle with grated cheese.
4. Bake at 200 degrees for 20 minutes.

Ready after 50 minutes

4 servings

Ingredients
- 1 large cubed butternut squash
- 2 tablespoons olive oil
- 1 1/2 cups red lentils
- 1 medium yellow onion, diced
- 2 teaspoons dried sage
- Himalayan salt and fresh cracked pepper
- 7 cups vegetable broth or water

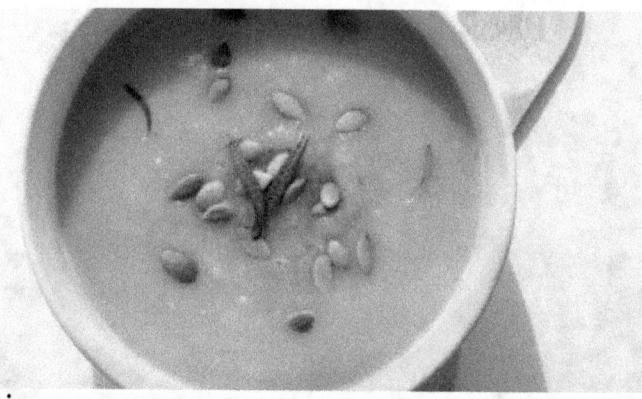

Preparation
1. Heat olive oil on an oven over medium heat. Add onions and cook them for about five minutes until they soften.
2. While stirring occasionally add squash and sage and cook for about 6 minutes. Add pepper, broth, salt, and lentils. Cook for 35 minutes on low heat while covered until the lentils and squash feel soft.
3. Allow them to cool and with your preferable method, puree the soup. Blend the soup using probably an immersion blender. Add liquid until the desired thickness is attained.
4. Serve preferably with chopped sage.

Ready after 1 hour

4 servings

Ingredients
- 1/4 cup shredded Parmesan
- 2 cloves garlic, minced
- 1 diced red pepper
- 2 tablespoons olive oil
- 1 whole spaghetti squash
- 1 carrot, shredded
- 1 zucchini, diced
- 16 ounces tomato sauce
- 1 tomato, diced
- 4 ounces shredded mozzarella cheese

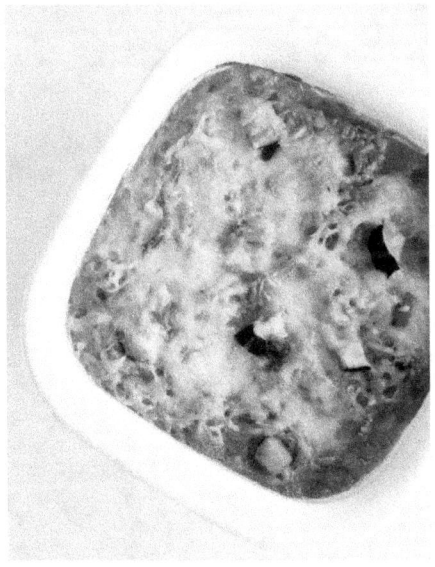

Preparation

1. Since you are to use your oven, it should be at about 350 degrees F so preheat it to that.
2. Take your spaghetti squash and cook it in a microwave until it's soft. This could take your ten minutes.
3. Adjust the heat to medium, and then add zucchini, carrots, garlic, oil, and pepper and cook.
4. Scoop the seeds of the squash out after cutting it into two. Peel it too to get the flesh separately. Take a casserole dish and inside it place the squash flesh.
5. Add diced tomato, a lot of the cheese, sauce, and the cooked veggies and make a good mixture.
6. Sprinkle with the remaining cheese the top of the mixture and cook until bubbling of the cheese is observed. Let it cool for a few minutes then serve.

Ready after 60 minutes

4 servings

Ingredients
- 3/4 teaspoon ground cumin
- 1 onion, diced
- 1 tablespoon olive oil
- 2 medium sweet potatoes, peeled and diced
- 1 can black beans, rinsed and drained
- 1 teaspoon minced garlic
- 1/2 teaspoon salt
- 4 cups veggie broth
- 1 can navy beans, rinsed and drained
- 2 tablespoons fresh lime juice
- 3/4 teaspoon ground coriander
- 1/2 teaspoon pepper

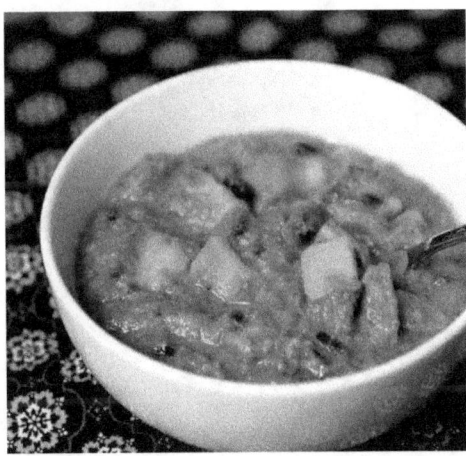

Preparation

1. Adjust the heat to medium heat then heat the oil in a pan. Add the onion, already chopped, and cook until they are soft. That needs around 15 minutes.
2. Make a mixture of cumin, coriander, pepper and salt. Add beans, vegetable broth and diced sweet potatoes. Boil while uncovered for about 25 minutes. This should be until the feel of the potatoes is tender.
3. Get ready the sweet potatoes and 3 cups of cooked beans. Using a hand blender, puree the remaining soup.
4. Get the reserved potatoes and beans back to cook for 15 minutes in the pot. If you have lemon juice, add it then season with pepper and salt.
5.

Ready after 50 minutes

4 servings

Ingredients
- Juice of 1/2 lemon
- 2 tablespoons coconut oil
- 4 minced cloves garlic, divided
- 1/4 cup low-sodium vegetable broth
- 1 thinly sliced small red chili
- 1 julienned large carrot
- 1 tablespoon minced ginger
- ½ stemmed, seeded and diced red bell pepper
- Coarse salt
- 2 tablespoons shelled pumpkin seeds
- 1 sliced divided red onion
- 2 tablespoons fresh cilantro leaves
- 2 cups cauliflower florets
- 2 cups broccoli florets

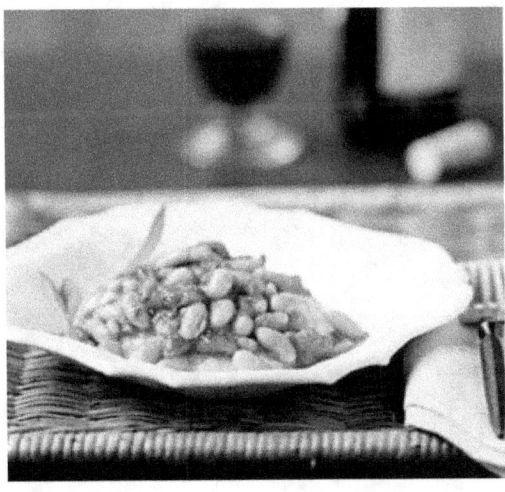

Preparation

1. Chop cauliflower florets until finely chopped in a food processor
2. Using your skillet, heat 1 tablespoon of coconut oil over medium heat. Add 2 minced garlic cloves and about half of the sliced red onion; then stir for about 8 minutes until tender.
3. Add cauliflower then using the coarse salt, season it.
4. Add in the vegetable broth and stir while steaming until broth evaporates leaving the cauliflower tender. Place it in a bowl and cover it.
5. Get the pan cleaned, and then use it to heat, over medium heat, one tablespoon oil.
6. Add half the red onion and cook for five minutes while stirring until it is tender. Add chili, ginger and garlic and cook for 60 seconds.
7. Add bell pepper, carrot and broccoli florets then cook for six minutes; that is, until they are tender.
8. Season with salt then add lemon juice after removing from heat.
9. Sprinkle with 1 tablespoon cilantro and a tablespoon of pumpkin seeds to serve.

SNACK

Celery chips

<u>Ready in 35 minutes</u>

<u>Servings: 5</u>

Ingredients
- ✓ 100g celery
- ✓ 2 tbsp. coconut oil
- ✓ Oregano
- ✓ Salt

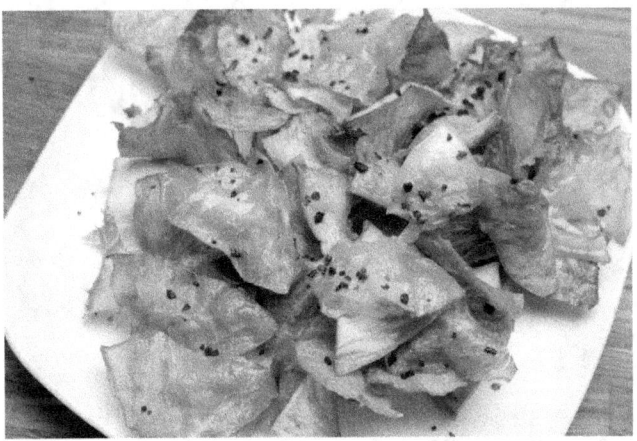

Preparation
1. Peel the celery, grate into thin slices with a mandolin or machine.
2. Spread them one by one on parchment paper and dry in a rotating oven for at least 30mn. Be careful not to blacken the celery: The oven door can also be opened a little to let the steam escape.
3. In a frying pan, heat enough oil (coco or classic) and add the celery slices so that they bathe, sprinkle with oregano and salt.

Chantilly cream and strawberries

<u>Ready in 2 minutes</u>

<u>Servings: 2</u>

Ingredients
- ✓ 40 g Raw Strawberries
- ✓ 50 ml Fresh liquid cream
- ✓ 1 tsp. sweetener
- ✓ Vanilla

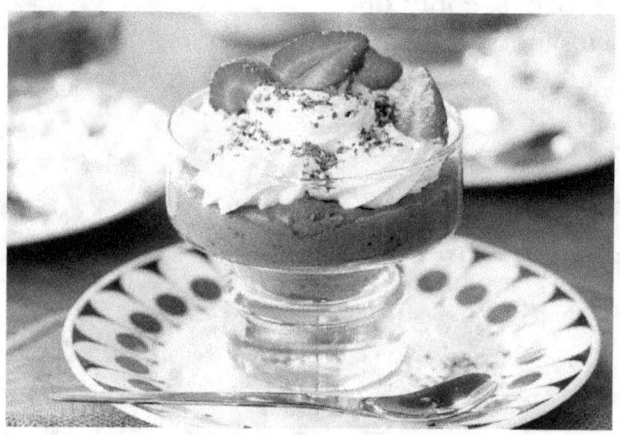

Preparation
1. Empty liquid cream into a siphon and add a few drops of sweetener and vanilla.
2. While closing the siphon, put the cartridge and shake the siphon 4 times and serve.

Creamy vanilla ice cream

Ready in 5 minutes

Servings: 5

Ingredients:
- ✓ 180g of ice
- ✓ 1 egg yolk
- ✓ 3 g of vanilla sugar
- ✓ 80g mascarpone
- ✓ 80ml whipping cream 30% fat
- ✓ Some fresh vanilla pod beans

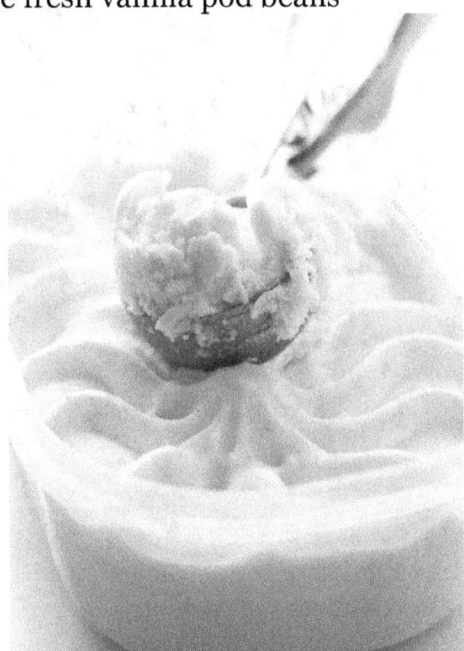

Preparation
1. Mix egg yolk with vanilla sugar and mascarpone and add the vanilla bean kernels. In a very cold bowl, beat the whipped cream.
2. Mix the Chantilly with the rest of the ingredients. Freeze for at least 4 hours.

<u>Ready in 25 minutes</u>

<u>Servings: 2</u>

Ingredients
- ✓ 11 g butter
- ✓ 15 g of chocolate
- ✓ 15 g of fresh cream
- ✓ ½ egg

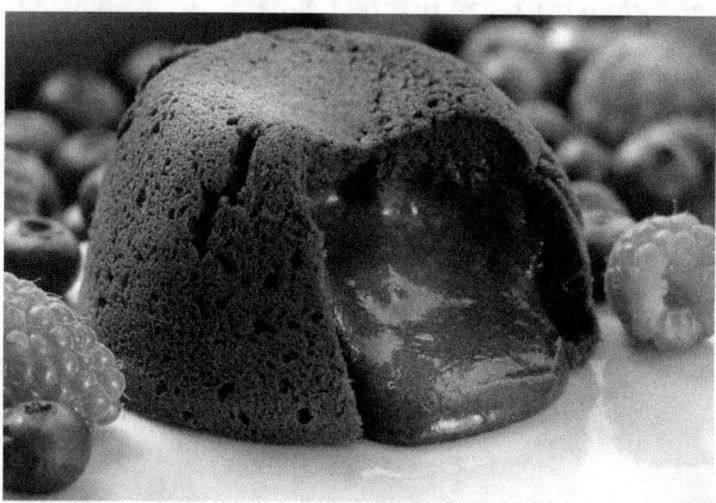

Preparation
1. Melt the chocolate with warm water, add the sweetener, cream, melted butter, egg yolk and snow-white.
2. Heat the oven to 200F. Cook the fondants on a baking tray for 10 minutes (the tops should form a crust).
3. Remove fondants from the oven.
4. Serve with caramel sauce and vanilla ice cream.

Ready in 15 minutes

Servings: 10

Ingredients
- ✓ 40g of fresh cream
- ✓ 62g of olive oil
- ✓ 25g of soy flour
- ✓ 40g almond powder
- ✓ 4g of yeast
- ✓ 1 egg
- ✓ 35g of dried tomatoes
- ✓ 60g of black olives

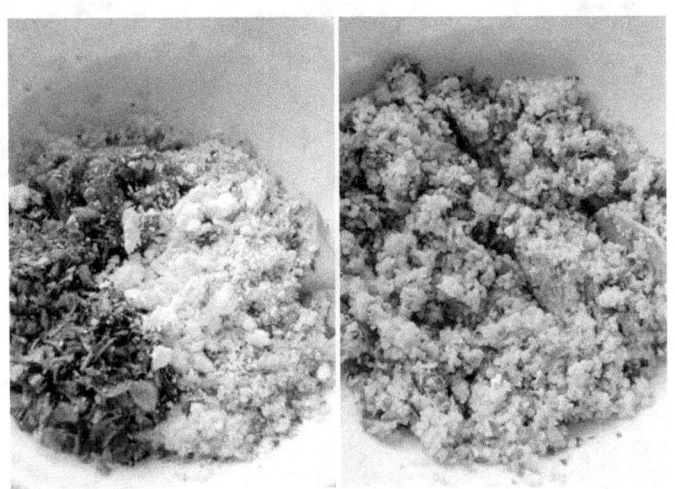

Preparation

Heat cream and oil together and let cool. In a bowl, combine the flour, almond powder, yeast and the egg. Then add the remaining oil and cream, dried tomatoes (mixed) and the olives (in small pieces) and mix the paste. Bake at 180 ° C for 15 minutes. If you use small fluted molds, you will get 20 mini-cakes.

<u>Ready in 20 minutes</u>

<u>Servings: 5</u>

Ingredients
- ✓ Mix of parsley and sorrel leaves, and 200g
- ✓ Beef stock, 1 liter
- ✓ Egg yolk,
- ✓ 100ml fraiche cream

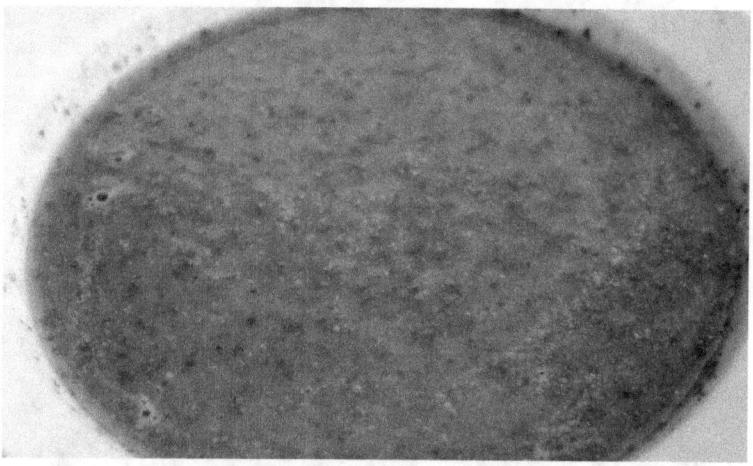

Preparation
3. Wash the leaves. Chop them in long strings until they look like large noodles.
4. Boil the beef stock. Add the leaves. Simmer for a minute or two.
5. Cool the broth for about 5 minutes.
6. Get about 2-3 ladles of the hot broth. Let it cool for another minute.
7. Mix the yolk and the fraiche cream in a cup.
8. Slowly add the yolk and fraiche cream mixture into the separated broth, whisk carefully and continuously to avoid coagulating the yolk.
9. Pour this mixture into the main pot of broth and the leaves. Mix well and serve immediately.

Ready in 25 minutes

Servings: 3

Ingredients
- ✓ ¾ Cup of Almond Flour
- ✓ 4 Tablespoons of Butter
- ✓ 2 Tablespoons of Sweetener
- ✓ 84g Pecans
- ✓ 4 Eggs
- ✓ ½ Tablespoon of Lemon Juice
- ✓ 9 Strawberries
- ✓ ½ Tablespoon of Vanilla Extract
- ✓ 1 1/2lbs of Cream Cheese
- ✓ ¼ Cup of Sour Cream

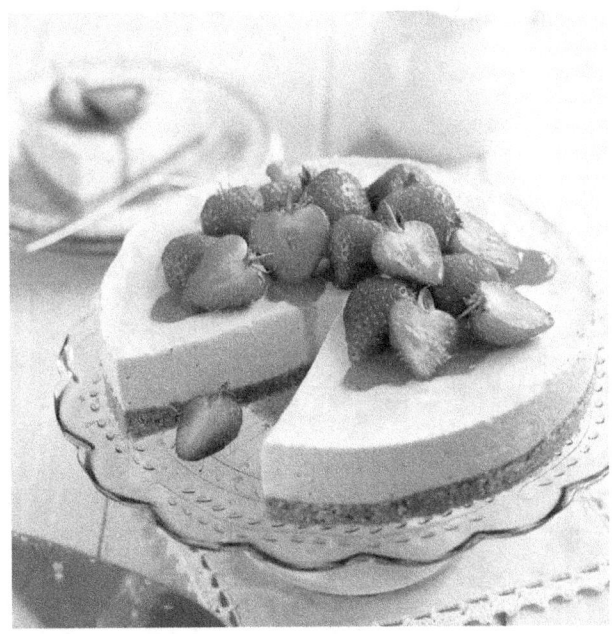

Method:
1. Pre-heat oven (700F)
2. Crush Pecans
3. Melt Butter in a saucepan and add flour, sweetener, and pecans
4. Mix until combined
5. Grease Spring form pan and line with the base (saucepan ingredients)
6. Cook until brown (5-6 minutes)
7. Combine filling ingredients with a whisk
8. Slice strawberries to line crust with
9. Pour filling on top of strawberries and crust
10. Bake in oven at 250 degrees for sixty-ninety minutes
11. Let cool when cooked, refrigerate and serve with cream

Ready in 1 hour

Servings: 5

Ingredients
- ✓ 1/3 cup coconut milk
- ✓ ½ cup dark chocolate
- ✓ 5 whole eggs
- ✓ 3 separated eggs
- ✓ ¼ cup coconut oil
- ✓ ¾ cup Almond meal
- ✓ 1 Teaspoon vanilla extract

Method:
1. In a bowl, add in the three egg white and beat it until stiff. Using the double boiler technique melt the dark chocolate.
2. In another bowl, add in the five eggs, the three yolks and keep mixing. To this add the coconut flour little by little.
3. Next, add in the coconut oil and melted chocolate and keep stirring in one direction. Fold in the egg whites into the mixture.
4. Add in the vanilla extract. Pre-heat your oven to 180 degrees Celsius. Grease the cake tin and line it with baking paper.
5. Pour the mixture into the cake tin. Bake in the oven for 40 minutes at 180 degrees Celsius. Allow the cake to cool before serving.

<u>Ready in 7 minutes</u>

<u>Servings: 5</u>

Ingredients
- ✓ 1 Strawberry
- ✓ 1/3 Cup of Whipping Cream (Heavy)
- ✓ 2 ½ grams of cocoa powder (unsweetened)
- ✓ 4 Drops of liquid sweetener
- ✓ 14g of whey powder (Chocolate)
- ✓ Chocolate Flakes

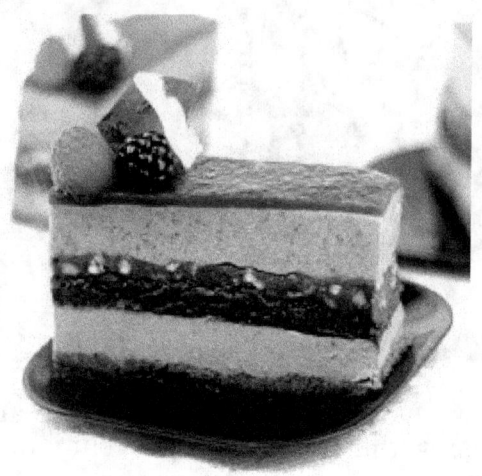

Method:
1. Measure the cream, sweetener, strawberry, powder and flakes into a mixing bowl
2. Mix for at least two minutes
3. Serve when mixture is stiff

Crusty fried cheddar bite

Ready in 20 minutes

Servings: 5

Ingredients
- ✓ Cheddar, 2 slices, 50 grams each
- ✓ Almond flour, 1 teaspoon
- ✓ Egg, whole, 1
- ✓ Flaxseed, ground, 1 teaspoon
- ✓ Hemp nuts, 1 teaspoon
- ✓ Olive oil, 1 tablespoon
- ✓ Salt and pepper to taste

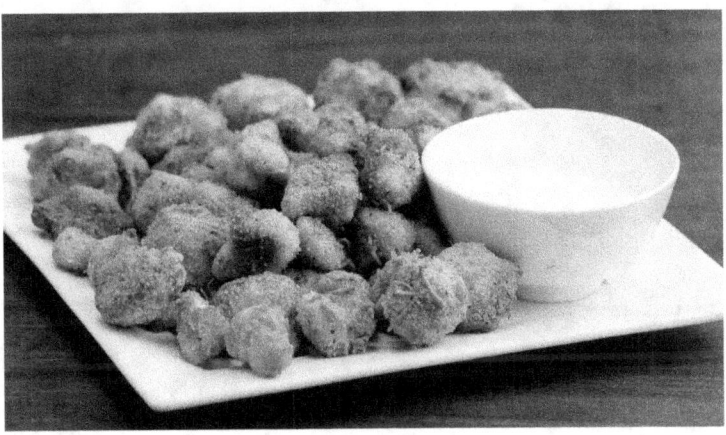

Preparations
1. Heat a frying pan over medium heat.
2. Add a tablespoon of olive oil.
3. Whisk the egg and add the salt and pepper.
4. Mix the ground flaxseed, hemp nuts and almond flour.
5. Coat the cheddar slices. Start with the egg mix, then with the dry.
6. Fry for 3 minutes on each side. Serve hot.

Conclusion

If you have never tried this diet before, it's your chance now to get a glimpse of the best weight loss diet. The other main advantages of these diet over other diets is that this diet is used to cure diseases such as infantile spasms, epilepsy, autism, brain tumors , Alzheimer's disease. Low-carb and ketogenic diets potentially bring several other benefits to the brain as compared to other diets.

Before You Go

If you liked this book you may like these other books from
Henry White

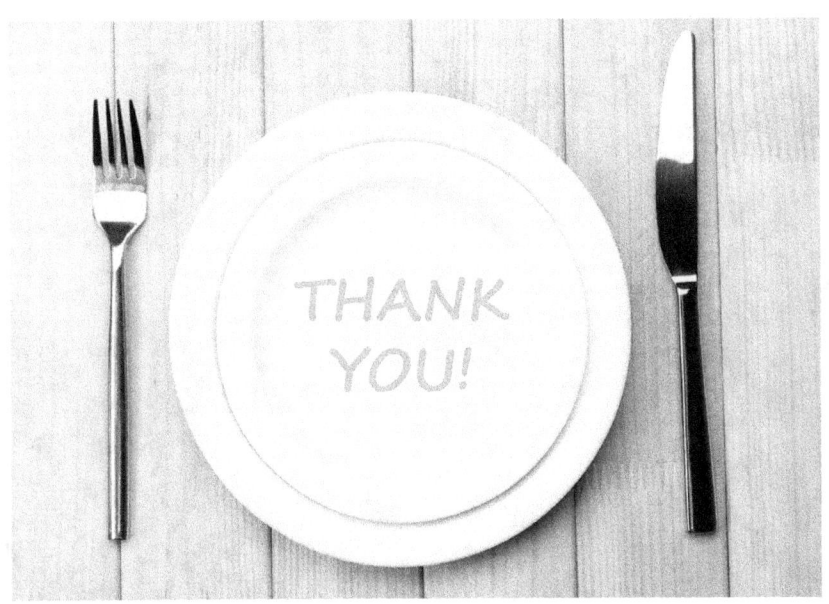

Did you enjoy this book?

I want to thank you for purchasing and reading this book. I really hope you got a lot out of it.

Can I ask a quick favor through?

If you enjoyed this book I would really appreciate ii if you could leave me an honest review on Amazon.

www.ingramcontent.com/pod-product-compliance
Lightning Source LLC
Chambersburg PA
CBHW062106280526
45788CB00003B/1359